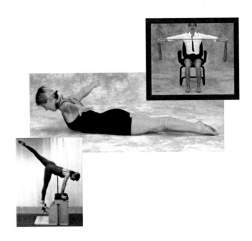

INTRODUCTION to TheraPilates® and Yoga
for Bone Building & Injuries

with
Sherri R. Betz, PT, GCS, PMA®-CPT

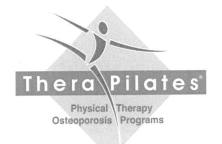

INSTRUCTOR BIOGRAPHY:

SHERRI BETZ, PT, DPT, GCS, CEEAA, PMA®-CPT is a 1991 graduate of the LSUMC School of Physical Therapy, a doctor of physical therapy, a Board Certified Geriatric Specialist, and a PMA® Certified Pilates Teacher. Sherri actually began her movement career as a national gymnastics competitor and as a group fitness instructor and personal trainer in the1980's. Inspired by the work of a physical therapist in one of the clubs where she trained, Sherri pursued a degree in physical therapy.

Her love of movement education has been integrated into her physical therapy practice at a rehabilitative level and at a fitness level. Utilization of Pilates methods, yoga, and Gyrotonic® with a specialty in the treatment of the pelvic girdle and manual therapy of the spine and pelvis are integral in her practice as a physical therapist.

Sherri was elected as the **Vice-President of the Pilates Method Alliance** and served on the PMA Board of Directors from 2003-2009. Sherri is the Chair of the PMA Research Committee and the Chair of the PMA Certification Board to protect the integrity of the credential and to improve the quality and safety of Pilates instruction.

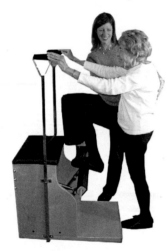

Selected to serve on the Board of Directors of **American Bone Health**, on the **FORE** (Foundation for Osteoporosis Research and Education) Professional Education Committee, on the **NOF** (National Osteoporosis Foundation) Exercise and Rehabilitation Advisory Council and as the Chair of the APTA Geriatric Section's **Bone Health Special Interest Group**, Sherri speaks internationally on behalf of these organizations on the topic of geriatric exercise, bone health and Pilates-based rehabilitation.

Sherri is passionately devoted to improving awareness about bone health through development of professional and consumer education as well as through promotion of low-cost community exercise programs for fit and frail older adults.

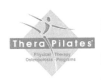

Safe Pilates for Bone Health
with Sherri Betz, PT, GCS, CEEAA, PMA®-CPT

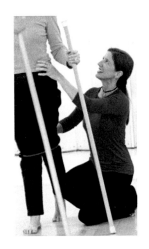

Osteoporosis is defined by low bone mass and micro-architectural deterioration of bone tissue leading to enhanced bone fragility and a consequent increase in fracture risk. (25% or greater bone loss)

3 Main Causes for Fracture in Bone:
1) Decreased bone mass or "Skeletal Fragility"
2) Impaired repair of the microdamage caused by normal wear and tear of bone, especially cancellous or trabecular bone
3) Falls

Bone is living dynamic; creating our blood cells"

"1 in 2 women & 1 in 4 men over age 50 will have an osteoporotic fracture in their lifetime

Osteopenia-Mildly reduced bone mass; a risk factor (10-20% bone loss)

Osteoblasts-Bone cells that function in building bone

Osteoclasts-Bone cells that function in breaking down old bone

Cortical Bone-Compact, contained in the long bones and outer layers of bone, 80% of skeletal mass, slow metabolism

Trabecular Bone-Cancellous or sponge-like, surface area is great, very metabolically active, high rate of turn over, 20% skeletal mass, makes bones light but strong. Contained in vertebral bodies and neck of femur.

Most common fracture sites:
Hip (Femoral Neck), Vertebral Bodies, Wrist and Ribs

Staggering Statisfics:
There are more deaths caused by osteoporosis than cancer of the cervix and breast combined. A woman's risk of hip fracture is equal to her combined risk of breast, uterus and ovarian cancer.

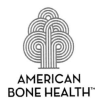

AMERICAN
BONE HEALTH™

www.therapilates.com

©TheraPilates® 2015

Bone Mineral Density:

Refers to the amount of mineral contained within a certain amount of bone: *1 gram of mineral for every square centimeter of bone = 1.0g/cm2*

Bone Mineral Density Testing:

Recommended that women get a baseline BMD test done on a **DEXA** machine at age 40 especially if risk factors are high

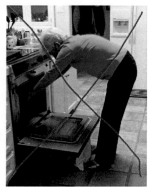

Interpretation of (DEXA) Bone Mineral Density Reports:

Tscore - Tells where the patient stands as compared to a young adult population for average peak bone mass

Zscore - Tells where the patient stands as compared to same age and sex normal population for average peak bone mass

For every 1 point drop in Standard Deviation below the mean, fracture risk doubles! -1=2x risk, -2=4x risk, -3=8x risk, -4=16x risk

FRACTURE PREVENTION:

1) Avoid all flexion, deep sidebending, and deep rotation of the spine
2) Sit up tall when coughing and sneezing - Do not bend forward!
3) Stand to the side of the oven and bend at the hip to reach into the oven
4) Keep your spine straight when putting on your shoes
5) Bend at the hips when you lean over the sink to brush your teeth or wash your face
6) Do not try to open heavy or stuck windows
7) Keep your spine elongated and straight when lifting heavyobjects especially from the floor
8) If an object cannot be lifted correctly in Neutral Spine alignment, don't lift it!
9) Avoid the Yoga Pigeon Stretch/Pilates Hip Stretch

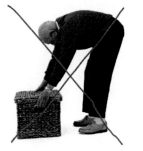
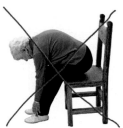
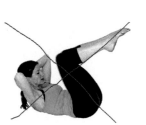
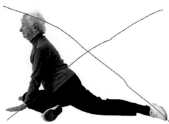

©TheraPilates® 2015

TREATMENT OPTIONS: *Medications, Nutrition, Exercise*

EXERCISE GUIDELINES:

1) Protect Spine from Fracture!! (First Priority!!)
2) Learn to Hip Hinge (Bend at hips instead of waist)
3) Learn Neutral Spine - up and down from floor to and from quadruped
4) Avoid all flexion (forward bending), deep sidebending and deep rotation (twisting) with Osteoporosis and Osteopenia of the spine
5) Practice Standing on 1 Leg (when you brush your teeth 2x per day!)
6) Learn to breathe with good rib movement and deep lower abdominal contraction
7) When all of the above are mastered begin bone building exercises

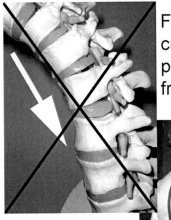

Forward Bending creates excessive pressure on the front of the spine

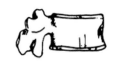

Normal Vertebra

Normal bone in spine (vertebra)

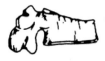

Wedge Fracture- usually from rounding the back

Wedge fracture

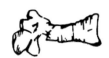

Crush Fracture- overhead lifting or spontaneous

Crush fracture

RED FLAGS:

1) Height loss of more than 1" (6cm or 2.4 inches predictive of vertebral compression fracture)
2) Previous Fracture
3) Family History (70% contributing factor)
4) Presence of Kyphosis (greater than 7cm occiput wall distance OWD is strongly predictive of fracture)

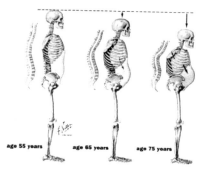

age 55 years   age 65 years   age 75 years

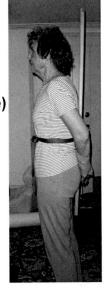

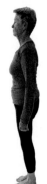

EXERCISE FOCUS:
Spinal Alignment and Elongation:

Standing Posture: Stand Tall with elongated spine

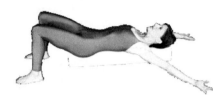

Thoracic Extension:

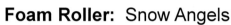

Foam Roller: Snow Angels

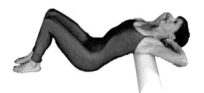

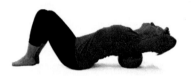

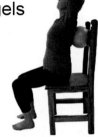

Foam Roller: Massage and Arching Stretches

8-9" Ball: Rolling up the spine, thoracic extension at individual vertebrae

Seated Thoracic Extension with Ball

Balance and Fall Prevention:

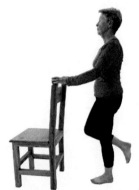

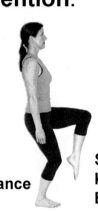

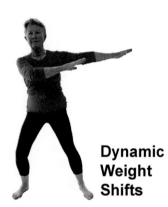

Single Leg Stance & Heel Raises

Single Leg Knee Bends

Dynamic Weight Shifts

Leg Strengthening:

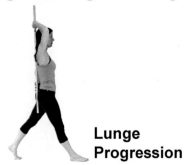

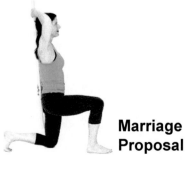

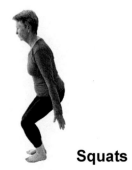

Lunge Progression

Marriage Proposal

Squats

REFERENCES:

1 Bansal, S., Katzman, W. B., & Giangregorio, L. M. (2014). Exercise for improving age-related hyper kyphotic posture: a systematic review. Arch Phys Med Rehabil, 95(1), 129-140.

2 Barker, KL. (2014). Physiotherapy Rehabilitation for Osteoporotic Vertebral Fracture (PROVE): study protocol for a randomised controlled trial.

3 Bird, M. L., & Fell, J. (2014). Positive long-term effects of Pilates exercise on the aged-related decline in balance and strength in older, community-dwelling men and women. J Aging Phys Act, 22(3), 342-347

4 Bone Heath and Osteoporosis-A Report of the Surgeon General. US Dept. of Health and Human Services, Public Health Services, Office of the Surgeon General, Rockville, MD; 2004

5 Briggs AM, et. al. Paraspinal muscle control in people with osteoporotic vertebral fracture. European SpineJournal. 2006 Nov.

6 Davis CM. Complementary Therapies in Rehabilitation, 2nd. Ed. Slack Publishing, 2004

7 Hu J, Zhao, Chen J, Fitzpatric J, Parpra B, Campbell TC. Bone density and characteristics in premenopausal and postmenopausal Chinese women. (Part of the China-Cornell Project) lifestyle character- Osteoporosis Int. 1994 Nov;4(6):288-97.

8 Lindsay R, et al. Risk of new vertebral fracture in the year following a fracture. JAMA. 2001 Jan17;285(3):320-3.

9 National Osteoporosis Foundation. America's Bone Health: The State of Osteoporosis and Low Bone Mass in Our Nation. Washington, DC: National Osteoporosis Foundation; 2002.

10 Pilates, JP. Return to Life Through Contrology. Pilates Method Alliance: Miami, FL, 2003 (originally published 1945), pg. 6.

11 Sinaki M (2013). Yoga spinal flexion positions and vertebral compression fracture in osteopenia or osteoporosis of spine: case series. Pain Pract, 13(1), 68-75.

12 Sinaki M, Mikkelsen, BA "Postmenopausal spinal osteoporosis: Flexion versus extension exercises." Arch Phys Med Rehab 1984; 65;593-596.

WEBSITES:

www.AmericanBoneHealth.org
www.FORE.org
www.NOF.org
www.OsteoFound.org
www.TheraPilates.com

Sherri R. Betz, PT, GCS, CEEAA
TheraPilates Physical Therapy Clinic
920-A 41st Avenue
Santa Cruz, CA 95062
831-476-3100
sherri@therapilates.com

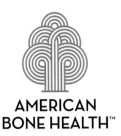

AMERICAN
BONE HEALTH™

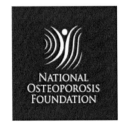

NATIONAL
OSTEOPOROSIS
FOUNDATION

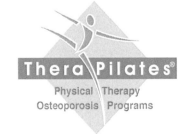

©TheraPilates® 2015

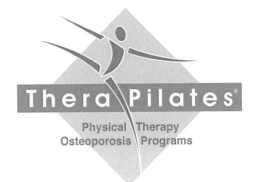

Thera Pilates®
Physical Therapy
Osteoporosis Programs

Posture Cues and Exercises

GOALS and SKILLS for *INTRODUCTION TO PILATES FOR BONE BUILDING AND INJURIES CLASS*

Class #1 – *Posture & Breathing* Skill Goals:
1. Breath with good rib movement and with abdominal wall firm. (page 12)
2. Be able to perform the hip hinge or "Chair Pose" with the Dowel continuously touching the 3 points of contact. (p. 13)
3. Establish your optimal postural alignment using the 7 Standing and Centering Cues with "relaxed" low back muscles. (pp. 14-15)

Class # 2 - *Leg Alignment* Skill Goals:
1. Keep arches lifted with 60% of weight on the outside of foot and 40% to the inside. When knees bend keep them aiming over the 4th and 5th toes no matter where the foot is pointing. (p. 14)
2. Practice heel raises with tennis ball between heels, then try on one leg. (p. 16)
2. Practice the 3-foot stride Marriage Proposal Lunge. (p. 18)
3. Practice the Single Leg Knee Bend. (Stand against the doorframe if you need support) (p. 17)

Class #3 - *Core Control* Skill Goals:
1. Transition to the floor in neutral spine and good leg alignment ideally using the Marriage Proposal Lunge transition (p. 19)
2. Quadruped weight shifts with neutral spine (pp. 19-20)
3. Side to Side and Pelvic Clock finding neutral with ease and relaxed low back muscles (pp. 22-23)
4. Bridging with spinal articulation and if possible stable pelvis at top with marching (p. 24)
5. Dip the Foot in the Pool- with no abdominal bulge, keeping pelvis and spine still (p. 25)
6. Bent Knee Opening and Assisted and Single Leg Circles- keeping pelvis and spine still (p. 26-28)
7. Sidelying and Clamshells with stable pelvis and low back relaxed (p. 29)
8. Prone Hip Extension with stable pelvis, knees straight and low back relaxed (p. 32)

Class #4 - **Shoulder Girdle Stability and Mobility Skill Goals:**
1. Good Spine and Rib Cage Alignment (pp. 14-15)
2. Practice Taut Towel Pulls with placement of the shoulder blades and collarbones on the rib cage (p. 34)
3. Placement of the humeral head posteriorly in the socket (using Towel p. 34)
4. Keeping the shoulder blades down and forward when reaching overhead
5. Aiming the socket of the shoulder upwards and wrapping the shoulder blade/arm pit around the ribcage when reaching overhead
6. Keeping the upper trapezius (neck muscles soft/relaxed when using the arm
7. Arms like a parenthesis especially in weight bearing
8. Pulling the shoulder blades wide and forward when in weightbearing of the upper extremities

Class #5 - Spine Mobility & Dynamic Stability Skill Goals:

1. Mobilize the mid thoracic spine on the 8" Massage Ball or Foam Roller regularly and remember to mount safely. (pp. 35-38)
2. Follow the mobilization with prone 3 part thoracic extension (p. 39)
3. Use a pillow under ribs and pelvis to protect your ribs with low bone density
4. Avoid endrange spine motions with low bone density
5. Practice Pelvic Clock and Side to Side to increase mobility of lumbar spine (pp. 22-23)
6. Practice Book Opening to increase mobility of thoracic spine (p. 41)
7. For advanced core control, practice Side Lift and Prone Pelvic Lift (pp. 31-33)

Class #6: Review and put it all together in one class!

To follow up from the 6 week series, the next step options are:

1. Repeat the Intro Class if you feel that you need more practice and feedback.

2. Go into the Level 2 Mon/Wed 8:45am or 10:00am twice weekly classes, or Tues 10am TheraPilates® for Bone Building Mat Classes held one time weekly.

3. Take the Level 2 Thursday 10:15am Yoga for Bone Building at TheraPilates®.

4. Take the Level 2 Pilates Mat Class at 11am on Saturdays at TheraPilates® (Drop-In $15, Package of 10 $120)

5. Take a Private Lesson from one of the TheraPilates® Pilates Teachers if you need more individual instruction or feedback on the exercises.

6. Book a physical therapy session with one of TheraPilates® licensed physical therapists if you have pain or injuries that did not get better with the classes.

7. Take a couple of private sessions to prepare for the TheraPilates® Reformer & Apparatus Classes: Limited to 5 People and classes occur Mon - Sat. Check the schedule online at www.therapilates.com

NOTE THAT "CLASSES" ARE GROUP SESSIONS AND "APPOINTMENTS" ARE EITHER PRIVATE PILATES OR PRIVATE PHYSICAL THERAPY 1 HOUR SESSIONS.

Feel free to call us at 831-476-3100 or email us at info@therapilates.com if you have any questions. Best of luck on your journey to vibrant health and movement!

Sincerely,
Sherri

Sherri Betz, PT, GCS, PMA®-CPT
Director of TheraPilates® Programs

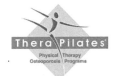

BREATHING TYPES: (Assess in Standing)
Diaphragmatic ☐   Upper Thoracic ☐   Lower Thoracic ☐
(Abdominal/Belly)   (Pump Handle)   (Costal)

Assess your dominant style of breathing by having a partner observing your breathing style preferably when you are unaware. Then take a deep breath to assess dominant style.

Assess your ability to use the following 3 breathing styles:
1. Are you able to take a *Diaphragmatic Breath* with expansion of low abdomen without movement of the pelvis or spine?
2. Are you able to take an *Upper Thoracic* (Pump Handle) breath with expansion of sternum and upper thoracic spine without neck tension or upper trapezius over-recruitment?
3. Are you able to take a *Lower Thoracic* (Costal) breath with expansion of lower ribs bilaterally without neck tension or upper trapezius over-recruitment?

RIB EXPANSION: (Assess in Standing)
Rest_____ ☐   Inhalation_____ ☐   Exhalation_____ ☐

To assess resting position, take a 2-3 deep breaths and exhale in a relaxed manner. Measure circumference at Xyphoid Process, T7, and Base of Scapulae at rest. Record score. Now, inhale as deeply as possible expanding the ribcage laterally into the arms/armpits. Record Inhalation score. Then exhale as fully as possible. Record Exhalation Score. Normal or Optimal is 2"expansion of lower ribs from rest position to full/deep inhalation.

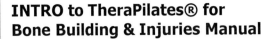

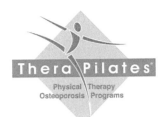

MAT WORK
Chair Pose in Neutral Spine

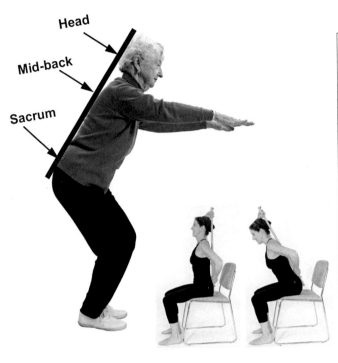

Head
Mid-back
Sacrum

BODY POSITION
Tie a 36 inch dowel or broomstick to your back with elastic band or straps around the chest underneath the armpits and around the waistline
Throughout the movement maintain contact with **head, mid-back,** and convex aspect of **sacrum** against dowel
Stand or sit in neutral spine with feet parallel to each other

MOVEMENT/BODY POSITION
Pretend that you are going to sit back in a chair (It is safer to actually have a chair behind you in case you lose your balance)
Aim your knees straight over the 2nd toe
Reach up as far as possible from fingertips to coccyx while keeping your shoulders down and back
Maintain lots of space between ears and shoulders
Elongate your spine from head to coccyx
Keep the abdominals drawn in
Hold for 3 deep costal breaths
Rest and repeat 2-3 times

WATCH FOR
Loss of neutral spine
Loss of contact with **head, midback** and convex aspect of **sacrum** against stick
Scapular elevation
Head looking up
Poor alignment of lower extremities

Relaxed Posture	Forced Correction	Best Correction
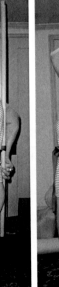	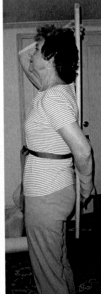	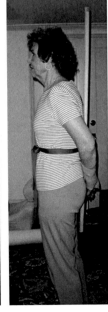

Sherri R. Betz, PT, GCS, CEEAA, PMA®-CPT
920-A 41st Avenue Santa Cruz, CA 95062
831.476.3100   www.TheraPilates.com

Ron Fletcher's
7 Standing and Centering Cues

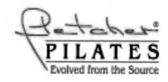

Foot Centers

Encourage   Avoid   Avoid

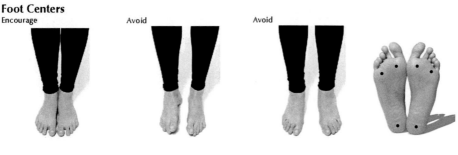

1. Tripod Foot Centers, find subtalar neutral, pronate and supinate, avoid collapsing of arch. 40% weight on inside of foot. 60% of weight on outside of foot.

Magnets

Encourage   Avoid

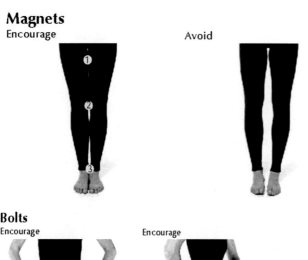

2. "Magnets" image between heels, shins and thighs (great for ankle control) Stand more often with feet together to activate postural muscles. Perform heel raises with feet together.

Bolts

Encourage   Encourage

Avoid   Avoid

3. Pelvic Bolts: Pubis to mid-sacrum Greater Trochanters Avoid tucking pelvis and tailbone under. Avoid arching pelvis and lifting tailbone up. Avoid squeezing buttocks. Keep pubis and tailbone level with back muscles relaxed.

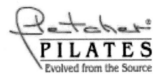

PILATES
Evolved from the Source

Girdle of Strength

Encourage   Avoid   Avoid

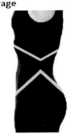 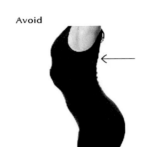 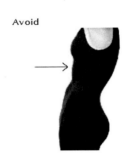

4. Girdle of Strength: Lift ribcage off pelvis especially from the sides. Keep ribcage centered over pelvis. Keep lumbar muscles relaxed.

Shoulder Girdle Placement

Encourage   Avoid

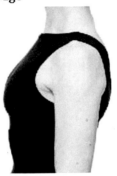 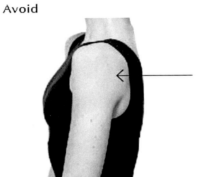

5. "Placement" of the shoulder blades and collarbones resting on the ribcage.

Head and Neck Placement

Encourage   Avoid   Avoid

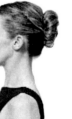 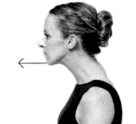 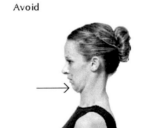

6. Draw the throat back and lift the ears up towards the ceiling. Lengthen the back of the neck.

Fletcher Percussive Breath™

Encourage   Encourage

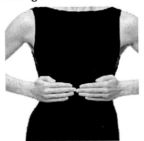 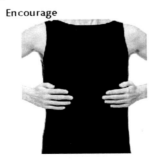

7. Percussive Breathing: Lateral Costal: supports core control

Diaphragmatic: relaxing

Upper lung: avoid, increases neck & shoulder tension

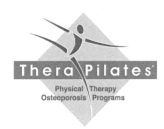

TENNIS BALL MASSAGE

Roll tennis ball longitudinally between metatarsals slowly from heel to ball of foot.

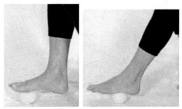
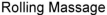
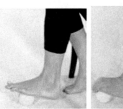
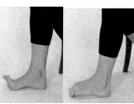

Rolling Massage   Parakeet/Wrap: MTP Flexion   Inch Worm

HEEL RAISE

Begin with tennis ball between ankles to practice subtalar neutral alignment.

Bilateral Correct Alignment with Tennis Ball Heel Lift   Unilateral Correct Alignment

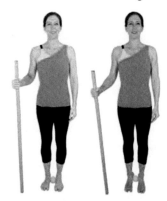
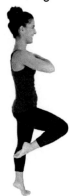

Remember:

1. Keep Ankle Subtalar Neutral Alignment
2. Keep Knee Straight
3. Keep Pelvis Level: avoid anterior translation, hiking, or shifting laterally
4. Maintain Rib to Pelvis Alignment: avoid rib shift anteriorly, laterally or posteriorly and torso lean
5. Maintain Shoulder Girdle Organization: avoid elevation, ab/adduction and keeps arms crossed

6. Maintain Head Alignment: avoid forward head or jutting of chin
7. Repeat 10x with good balance: avoid touching legs together, touching lifted foot to floor, excessive torso movement, hopping or flailing arms
8. May use chair back rest and or cane for balance assistance. Strongly encourage students to attempt exercise without assistive devices (float hand 2" off of chair back rest or hold dowel/can 2" off floor for safety)

Sherri R. Betz, PT, GCS, CEEAA, PMA®-CPT
920-A 41st Avenue Santa Cruz, CA 95062
831.476.3100   www.TheraPilates.com

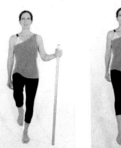

Start

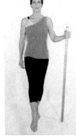

Flexion

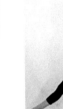

Bent Standing Leg

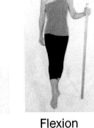

Abduction   Extension

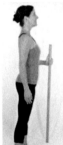 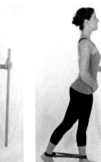

Resistance Bands

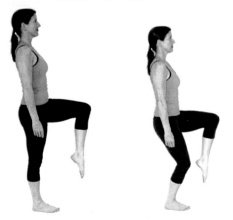

Single Leg Knee Bends

Sherri R. Betz, PT, GCS, CEEAA, PMA®-CPT
920-A 41st Avenue Santa Cruz, CA 95062
831.476.3100 www.TheraPilates.com

MAT WORK
Balance Series

BODY POSITION
Standing
Send all your weight to your left foot
Lift your right knee and hip to a 90
   degree angle
Left foot pointed straight ahead and
   aligned with patella
Maintain neutral spine
Draw scapulae towards waist
Lift ribs away from pelvis
Move head towards the ceiling to
   lengthen cervical spine
Keep pelvis level

MOVEMENT/BREATHING
Inhale
Exhale and send your right leg forward
   until the knee is straight
Inhale and bend the knee, returning to
   center
Exhale send your right leg to the side
   until the knee is straight
Inhale and bend the knee, returning to
   center
Exhale and send your leg back until
   the knee is straight
Inhale and bend the knee, returning to
   center
Repeat sequence 3 times

VARIATIONS
1) Hold a chair back or stick for
   support
2) Do the whole series with the
   standing leg bent
3) Small Knee Bends of the stance
   leg
4) Stand on unstable surface

WATCH FOR
Anterior or posterior pelvic tilting
Excessive lumbar extension
Dropping pelvis on one side
Bending stance leg
Scapular elevation
Foot pronation
Knee valgus

MAT WORK
Marriage Proposal Lunges

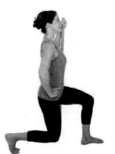

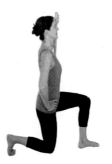

3 Foot Stride   **Heel Raise**   **Back Knee**   **Front Knee**

1   2   3   4

1/2 Lunge   **3/4 Lunge**   **Full Lunge**

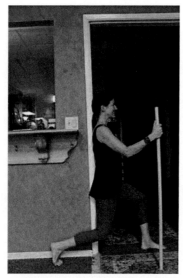

Modification against doorframe

BODY POSITION
Hold or tie a 48-inch dowel or broomstick against your back with elastic band or straps around the chest underneath the armpits and around the waistline.

Throughout the move-ment maintain contact with **head, mid-back**, and convex aspect of **sacrum** against dowel.

Stand in neutral spine with feet parallel to each other

MOVEMENT
1) Step 3 feet forward in parallel alignment.
2) Lift and lower back heel stretching the calf and hip flexor of the back leg.
3) Perform a small "secret" knee bend of the back knee keeping pelvis level and torso perfectly still. Avoid dropping the pelvis of the back leg.
4) Now keep the back knee straight and bend the front knee slightly without moving the torso forward.
5) Then perform a 1/4 bend straight down and back up.
   Progress to 1/2, 3/4 and Full by touching the knee to the floor (only if well-controlled and not painful.
6) Repeat with opposite leg forward.

WATCH FOR
Loss of neutral spine
Dropping pelvis or rounding back
Leaning trunk forward
Scapular elevation
Knee moving forward past toes
Foot pronating
Collapsing Ankle
Poor alignment of lower extremities
Short stride length

Sherri R. Betz, PT
920-A 41st Avenue Santa Cruz, CA 95062
831.476.3100 www.TheraPilates.com

18

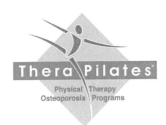

MAT WORK
Transitions in Neutral Spine

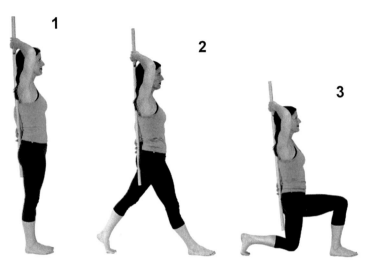

1 2 3

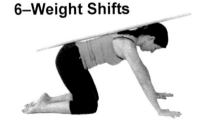

4

5-Pregnant Cat Breathing

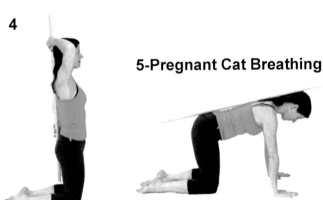

6–Weight Shifts

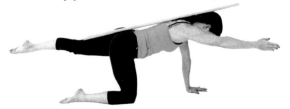

7-Opposite Shld Flex/Hip Ext

BODY POSITION
1) Hold or tie a 36 inch dowel or broomstick against your back with elastic band or straps around the chest underneath the armpits and around the waistline.
Throughout the movement maintain contact with **head, mid-back**, and convex aspect of **sacrum** against dowel.
Stand in neutral spine with feet parallel to each other

MOVEMENT
2) Step 3 feet forward in parallel alignment.
3) "Marriage Proposal" Lunge: Bend your knees and descend as if you are sliding down a wall. Aim your knees straight over the 2nd toe.
4) Bring the front knee back to a tall kneeling position without moving the spine or pelvis.
5) Sit back towards your heels.
6) Move to quadruped balancing the dowel on your back.
7) Reach opposite arm and leg up without losing the neutral spine position.
8) Reverse the positions and return to standing.
Repeat with opposite leg forward.

WATCH FOR
Loss of neutral spine
Loss of contact with **head, mid-back** and convex aspect of sacrum against stick
Bending trunk forward
Scapular elevation
Head looking up
Knee moving forward past toes
Foot pronating
Poor alignment of lower extremities

Sherri R. Betz, PT, GCS, CEEAA, PMA®-CPT
920-A 41st Avenue Santa Cruz, CA 95062
831.476.3100   www.TheraPilates.com

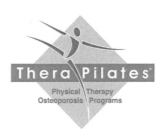

TheraPilates®
Physical Therapy
Osteoporosis Programs

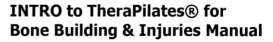
MAT WORK
Neutral Spine in Quadruped

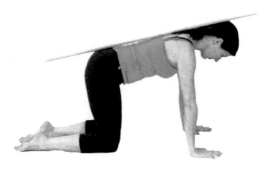

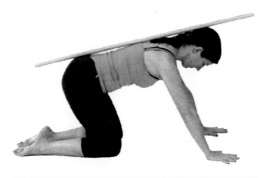

Quadruped Weight Shifts

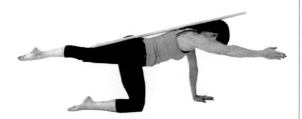

Opposite Shld Flex/Hip Ext

SETUP
Quadruped with shoulders over hands and hips over knees.

Pelvis and head in neutral position, spine in neutral curves, scapulae depressed, axial elongation.

Place dowel over spine in contact with head, mid-thoracic spine and sacrum

MOVEMENT / BREATHING
Inhale to prepare, expanding lower ribs postero-laterally, allowing abdomen to gently expand as well.

Exhale, moving one shoulder into flexion, reaching the arm forward, while moving opposite hip into extension, reaching the leg back — lengthening into axial elongation and keeping ribs engaged with pelvis.

Inhale, returning to quadruped, again lengthening into axial elongation and maintaining neutral pelvis and spinal curves. Repeat with other arm and leg

VARIATION
Lift one limb at a time

Lift same arm and leg with minimal hip or shoulder rotation

Props:

Hands and/or knees may be on rotating disks, foam rollers, balance boards, gym balls and any combination thereof.

Another option is to be quadruped over gym ball (ball under trunk)

CUEING
Axial elongation

Scapular depression and abduction

Integration of ribs with pelvis

WATCH FOR
Loss of axial length or neutral spine

Dropping into cervical or lumbar extension especially at L3

Scapular "winging" and elevation

Loss of abdominal support

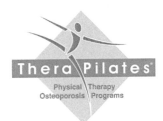

MAT WORK
Shoulder/Thoracic
Stretch

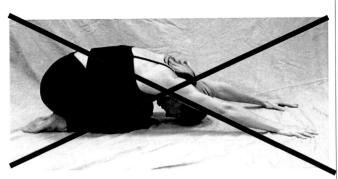

Shoulder Stretch (1/2 Down Dog)

BODY POSITION
  Start in all 4's quadruped

MOVEMENT/BREATHING
  Start in quadruped
  Keep hips directly over knees
  Walk hands forward until you feel a
    shoulder and body stretch
  Plant hands firmly on the floor
  Draw in the abdominals and send the
    outside of your armpits toward the
    floor
  Breath deeply and slowly into your
    lower lungs
  Imagine breathing directly into your
    low back
  Breath deeply and slowly and hold for
    up to 90 seconds

WATCH FOR
  Sagging of the ribs
  Shoulders moving towards ears
  Excessive lumbar extension or flexion
  Loss of abdominal support
  Hips sagging into hyperextension

Prayer Stretch (Child's Pose)
Avoid rounding your back.
Keep head off floor.
OK if knees are wide and ribs
are not pressing into thighs.

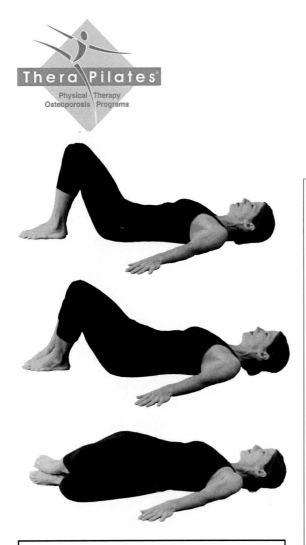

BASIC: With Feet Down

MAT WORK
Side to Side
(Gentle Lumbar Mobilization)

BODY POSITION
Start supine in neutral pelvis and spine.
Knees bent, heels about 12" away from buttocks.
Feet hip width apart.

MOVEMENT/BREATHING
Inhale to rotate pelvis and knees together to the left.
Rotate only as far as you can keep back of ribcage and shoulder blades on the mat.
Keep ribcage still by keeping back of lowest ribs on the mat.
Lengthen top of left pelvis away from lowest ribs for a gentle stretch.
Exhale rotating sequentially from the ribcage to the pelvis back to the starting position.

VARIATION
ADVANCED: Begin with knees bent 90 deg, hips above knees in a "table top" position.
Inhale to rotate pelvis and knees together to the left.
Rotate only as far as you can keep back of ribcage and shoulder blades on the mat.
Keep ribcage still by keeping back of lowest ribs on the mat.
Lengthen top of left pelvis away from lowest ribs for a gentle stretch.
Exhale rotating sequentially from the ribcage to the pelvis back to the starting position.

WATCH FOR
Flaring of ribs
Hyperextension or pain in lumbar spine
Lifting of opposite shoulder blade
Overflow of tension to the neck and shoulders
Pressing head into mat

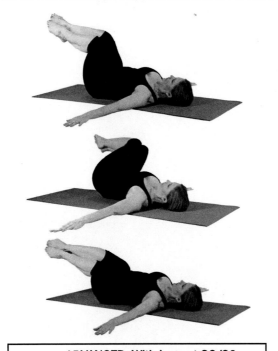

ADVANCED: With Legs at 90/90

Sherri R. Betz, PT, GCS, CEEAA, PMA®-CPT
920-A 41st Avenue Santa Cruz, CA 95062
831.476.3100   www.TheraPilates.com

22

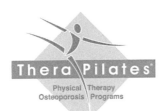

MAT WORK
Pelvic Clock
(Gentle Lumbar Mobilization)

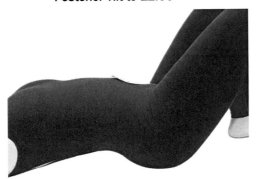

Posterior Tilt to 12:00

Antterior Tilt to 6:00

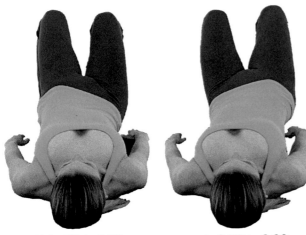

Right Tilt to 9:00   Left Tilt to 3:00

BODY POSITION
Start supine in neutral pelvis and spine.
Knees bent, heels about 12" away from buttocks.
Feet hip width apart.

MOVEMENT/BREATHING
12:00 Posterior Tilt:
Inhale to lengthen the spine.
Exhale to roll pelvis backward, drawing pubic bone towards the sternum. Low back will come closer to the floor. Keep buttocks relaxed.

6:00 Anterior Tilt:
Inhale to roll pelvis forward, sending pubic bone away from sternum. Low back will move away from floor. Exhale to return to neutral. Keep ribcage still by keeping back of lowest ribs on the mat.

9:00 Right Tilt:
Inhale to lengthen the spine.
Exhale to roll pelvis to the right, as if a marble is on your low belly and it would roll to the right.. Keep right buttock down on the mat. Keep ribcage still by keeping back of lowest ribs on the mat. Imagine that the legs are between 2 panes of glass and the knees will shift slightly forward and backward.

3:00 Left Tilt:
Inhale to lengthen the spine.
Exhale to roll pelvis to the left, as if a marble is on your low belly and it would roll to the left.. Keep right buttock down on the mat. Keep ribcage still by keeping back of lowest ribs on the mat.

WATCH FOR
Flaring of ribs
Hyperextension or pain in lumbar spine
Swaying of knees from side to side
Lifting of pelvis completely off the mat
Overflow of tension to neck and shoulders

TheraPilates®
Physical Therapy
Osteoporosis Programs

MAT WORK
Bridging

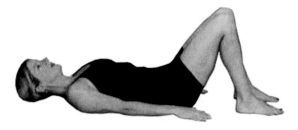

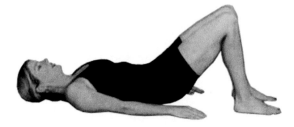

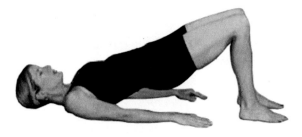

BODY POSITION
Lie supine.
Do not prop head and neck with pillows or a wedge unless a severe kyphosis or forward head is present.
Begin in neutral spine.

MOVEMENT/BREATHING
Inhale to lengthen the spine.
As you exhale, begin by drawing your pubic bone towards the sternum, aim your coccyx toward the ceiling, bring your pubic bone toward your sternum and lift each vertebrae off the mat one at a time until you are standing just between your scapulae (shoulder blades).
Inhale while you are up at the top. Send your knees far away from you, elongating your spine as much as possible.
Exhale and soften your sternum, sending it toward your pelvis
Keep your abdominals drawn in and lower each vertebrae down like a string of pearls.
Emphasize the placement of the low back onto the floor or the practitioner's hand.
Inhale and release the pelvis to neutral.

Marching Variation: Place dowel over pelvis, Keep pelvis level and lift one knee alternating 5 times each leg.

WATCH FOR
Cervical spine position
Raising the buttocks too high
Going up too high on the shoulders and neck
Losing posterior tilt
Ribs jutting up towards the ceiling
Dropping Pelvis on one side with Marching Variation

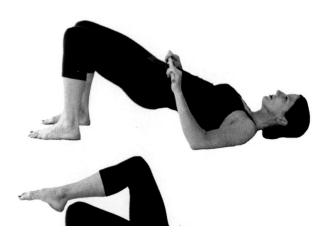

MAT WORK
Dip Foot in the Pool

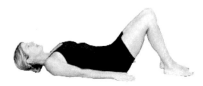

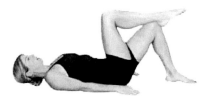

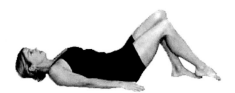

Basic Variation

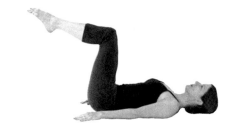

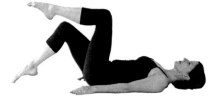

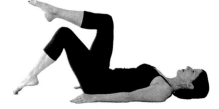

Advanced Variation

BODY POSITION
Lie supine propping head and neck with pillows or a wedge if an increased kyphosis or forward head is present
Maintain neutral spine

BASIC VARIATION: MOVEMENT/ BREATHING
Inhale to lengthen the spine.
Exhale as you lift your knee toward the ceiling until the shin is parallel to the floor.
Inhale when the knee is over the hip.
Exhale and point your toe, touch your foot to the floor as if you are touching the top of an egg.
Inhale
Exhale and bring your knee back to the starting position.

INTERMEDIATE VARIATION: MOVEMENT/BREATHING
Inhale to lower the foot to floor.
Exhale to lift the leg back to the tabletop position.

ADVANCED VARIATION:
keeping abdominal wall firm and spine and pelvis perfectly still starting with legs up at 90/90 Table Top Position in Neutral or Flat Back.
Inhale to touch the foot to the floor keeping knees at 90 degree angles.
Exhale to lift leg back to starting position.

WATCH FOR
Flaring of the ribs
Loss of neutral spine
Pelvis tilting

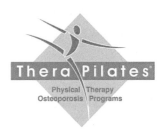

MAT WORK
Bent Knee Opening

Basic: Feet Down	Advanced: Legs Up in 90-90

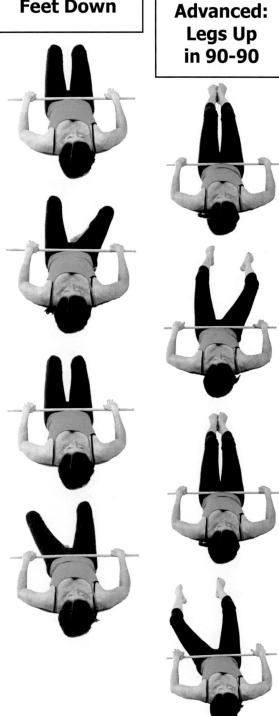

BODY POSITION

Lie supine propping head and neck with pillows or a wedge if an increased kyphosis or forward head is present. Knees bent and feet together. Maintain neutral spine.

MOVEMENT/BREATHING
BASIC VARIATION

Inhale
Exhale as you allow your right knee to drop away from you keeping pelvis still
Inhale
Exhale and bring your knee back to the starting position

ADVANCED VARIATION

Start with legs in table top position
Inhale as you allow your right leg to lower out to side, keeping right shin parallel to left shin.
Exhale to bring leg back to start position.
Repeat 5x each side.

WATCH FOR

Flaring of the ribs
Rotation of pelvis
Bulging of low belly
Loss of neutral spine

Sherri R. Betz, PT, GCS, CEEAA, PMA®-CPT
920-A 41st Avenue Santa Cruz, CA 95062
831.476.3100   www.TheraPilates.com

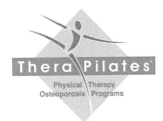
TheraPilates®
Physical Therapy
Osteoporosis Programs

MAT WORK
Assisted Hip Circles

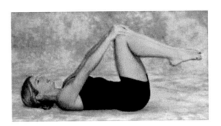

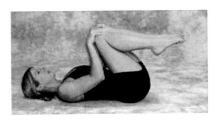

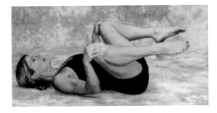

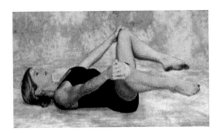

BODY POSITION
Lie supine propping head and neck with pillows or a wedge if an increased kyphosis or forward head is present. Maintain neutral spine.

MOVEMENT/BREATHING
Inhale as you passively bring your knees toward you
Exhale as you circle your knees outward and away from you

WATCH FOR
Loss of neutral spine
Rocking of pelvis

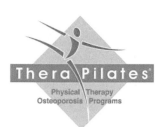

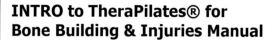

MAT WORK
Modified Hip Circles

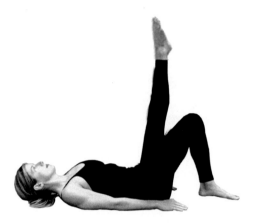

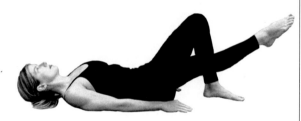

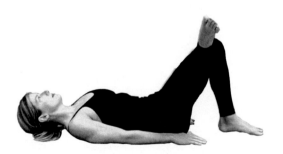

BODY POSITION
Supine
Hands with palms down, arms at sides
Shoulders depressed
Feet are plantarflexed with one knee
  extended or partially flexed and one
  knee bent with foot on mat
Hips: one extended, one flexed
Head / neck in neutral
Pelvis in neutral

MOVEMENT/BREATHING
Circumduct the raised leg
Inhale with the leg close to the trunk
Exhale with the leg away from the trunk
Pelvis and spine remain neutral
throughout the leg circle

VARIATIONS
Decrease the size of the circle
Increase the size of the circle
Bend knee of lifted leg

CUEING
Support the head and neck in the
  direction of axial length
Guide the shoulders toward depression
  and abduction
Guide the lower ribs toward the pelvis
Place hands on low belly to monitor
  movement of pelvis
Aim sit bone of raised leg toward
opposite foot, keeping waistline long

WATCH FOR
Either PSIS lifting off floor
Losing neutral spine /
pelvis Flaring ribs
Rotation of Pelvis

Sherri R. Betz, PT, GCS, CEEAA, PMA®-CPT
920-A 41st Avenue Santa Cruz, CA 95062
831.476.3100 www.TheraPilates.com

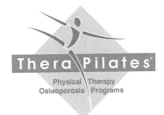

MAT WORK
Sidelying & Clamshells

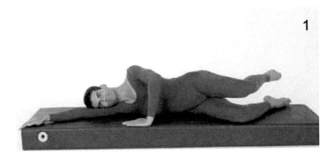

1

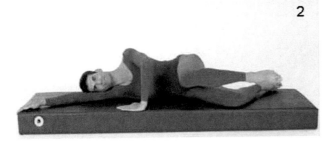

2

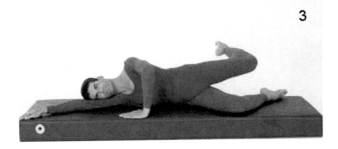

3

BODY POSITION
Side-lying on mat, head resting on pillow or lower arm outstretched overhead. Hand of upper arm on floor in front of rib cage.
The top hip should be directly over the bottom hip, waist lifted from the floor, pelvis/spine/head in neutral.
Pelvis and legs stacked on floor with hips and knees bent. Top leg lifted until parallel with floor. Imagine that the head, mid-back and buttocks are against a wall at the edge of a mat.

MOVEMENT / BREATHING
Sidekick: Inhale, move the top leg forward into hip flexion, maintaining neutral pelvis position.
Exhale, move the leg into hip extension, maintain neutral pelvis position.

VARIATIONS
1) **Clam shells:** Keep feet together and just lift knee, rotating the top hip, pointing knee towards the ceiling.
2) **Fire Hydrant:** Lift whole leg up with knee bent to 90 degree angle

CUEING
Keep the spine long and abdominal wall drawn in.
Keep shoulders down and back.
Keep the lower ribs aligned with pelvis .

WATCH FOR
Trunk flexion, extension, or rotation
Ribs sagging towards floor
Loss of axial length
Rocking of the pelvis

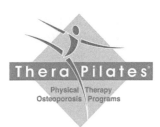

MAT WORK
Sidekick

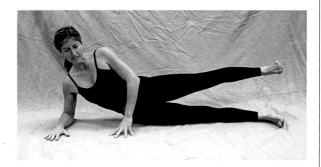

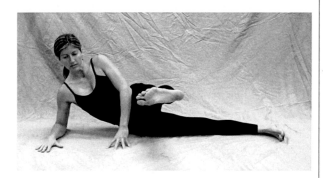

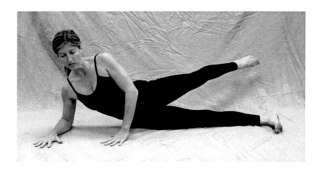

BODY POSITION
Side-lying on mat, up on elbow, with
with shoulder aligned over elbow, hand of
upper arm on floor in front of rib cage
The top hip should be directly over the
bottom hip, waist lifted from the floor,
pelvis/spine/head in neutral
Legs outstretched on floor with hips
in neutral, and feet flexed.
Top leg lifted until parallel with floor

MOVEMENT / BREATHING
Sidekick: Inhale, move the top leg forward
into hip flexion, foot flexed,
maintain neutral pelvis position
Exhale, move the leg into hip extension,
foot pointed, maintain neutral
pelvis position

VARIATION
1) Small Circles: Circle top leg 10 times in
each direction, using small pulsing
breaths
2) Bicycle: Bending top knee, move top
leg forward into hip flexion and
gradually into knee extension. When
leg is straight in front, sweep leg
backwards to full hip extension.
Repeat 5 x each side.
3) Bottom knee bent to 90 degrees
perform any of the above movements
with the bottom knee bent to add
stability.

CUEING
Keep head and throat pulled back in
direction of axial length
Draw the shoulders toward
depression and abduction
Draw the lower ribs toward the pelvis

WATCH FOR
Trunk flexion, extension, or rotation
Ribs sagging towards floor
Loss of axial length

MAT WORK
Sidelift

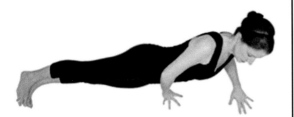

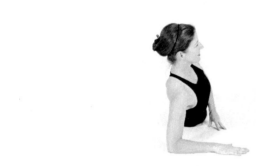

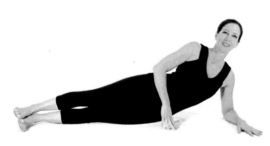

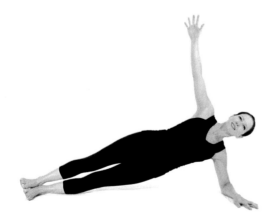

BODY POSITION
Sidelying

Spine in Neutral

Elbow placed just under the shoulder

Stack shoulders, hips, knees and ankles

Maintain a straight postural alignment as if you are standing up or against a wall

Dorsiflex ankles keeping ankle in a neutral position keeping outer ankle bone from touching the floor

Knees straight

Ribs lifted to form a triangle under the armpit

Bottom shoulder depressed away from ear

MOVEMENT/BREATHING
Inhale to prepare

Exhale as hips lift off floor

Inhale to release back to starting position

VARIATIONS
Regression: Use top hand for assistance

Regression: Just do a Rib Lift without lifting the hips

Regression: Bend bottom knee, keeping thighs in alignment

Progression: Raise top hand to ceiling, behind head or at waist or progress to the Star

CUEING
Keep the head and neck lengthened

Guide the bottom shoulder toward depression and abduction

Lift the lower ribs gently upwards

Lift the pelvis up to assist the client in initiating the movement

Imagine (or actually place) your head, mid-back and tailbone against a wall

WATCH FOR
Sagging of lowest ribs

Shoulder elevating towards ear

Supination of feet

Lateral Malleolus touching the floor

Pointing of toes

Stepping on the bottom foot

Slipping of the feet especially if in socks-- indicates poor core control

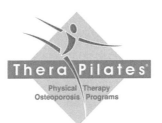

MAT WORK
Hip Extension

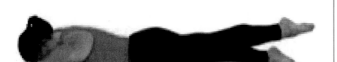

**Pelvis Neutral/Low Back Relaxed:
Hip Extension with Knee Straight**

BODY POSITION
Prone: Elongate pelvis away from the ribcage. Hands under forehead.
Slide scapula down and back with back of neck lengthened.

MOVEMENT/BREATHING
Inhale to prepare
Exhale as you reach the right leg long and lift the thigh 1-2", keeping the knee straight.
Press the pelvic bones into the mat.
Inhale to lower the leg.
Repeat on both sides 10x.

PROGRESSIONS
Pulse the leg 20x quickly.
Add the opposite arm reaching up while drawing the shoulder blade down.

WATCH FOR
With Leg Raise:
Extension or arching of lumbar spine
Back, neck, or shoulder pain
Pubic bone lifting
Tailbone lifting
Hip Hiking
Knee bending
Pelvis rotating

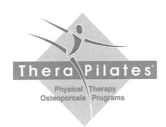

MAT WORK
Prone Pelvic Lift

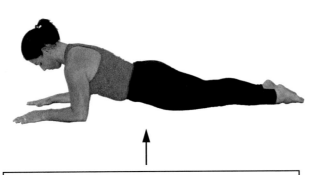

**Pubis lifted no more than 1" off mat.
Pelvis in strong posterior tilt.**

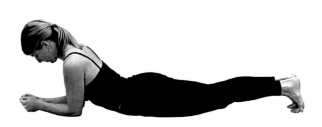

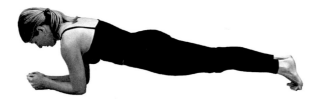

BODY POSITION
Prone on elbows
Shoulders over elbows
Draw scapulae towards waist
Pubis pressed into mat
Lift sternum to ceiling

MOVEMENT/BREATHING
Inhale to prepare
Exhale and draw your pubic bone
  towards your sternum pressing it into
  the mat, then lifiting it up no more
  than 1". You should be feeling a deep
  abdominal contraction
Send your coccyx toward your feet
without squeening the glutes.
Continue to lift until ears, shoulders,
  hips and knees are aligned
Inhale and release slowly back to
  starting position

VARIATION
  1) Knees straight, plank position
  2) Keep both feet and knees on the
     floor

WATCH FOR
Scapulae moving up towards ears
Chest sinking down
Winging scapulae
Sagging of the ribs
Shoulders moving towards ears
Excessive lumbar extension
Lifting coccyx toward ceiling with
  inappropriate use of Iliopsoas
  muscle
Loss of abdominal contraction
Loss of support from core musculature
Hips sagging into hyperextension

***Very good preparation
for push- ups!!*

Sherri R. Betz, PT, GCS, CEEAA, PMA®-CPT
920-A 41st Avenue Santa Cruz, CA 95062
831.476.3100 www.TheraPilates.com

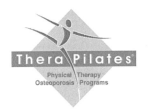

MAT WORK
Fletcher® Towelwork

Shoulder Setting: Preparation for all upper body work:

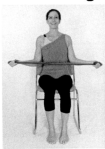

Seated

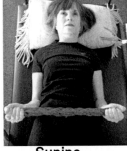

Supine

Hold Towel about 20" apart palms up. Imagine that you are holding a serving tray. Sit tall in optimal postural alignment. Inhale to widen collarbones and roll humeral heads back and down in the sockets. Exhale and pull Towel until it is gently taut while maintaining the humeral head and scapular position. Open collarbones. Avoid "squeezing" or adducting scapula. Repeat 10x.

Taut Towel Pulls:

Hold towel at double the distance of your shoulder girdle with palms down and back of the wrists flat. Elbows are slightly bent with arms in a parenthesis shape. Keep shoulders down and inhale to lengthen the spine then exhale and pull the towel from your back. Keep your neck relaxed and wrists firm. Repeat 5x with the towel in front of your hips, 5x with the towel at your collarbone height and 5x with the towel overhead. Now raise your arms to the overhead position, by initiating the lift of your arm from your back. Draw your armpit down and forward to lift. Hold the towel over the crown of your head, turn your armpits to face forward and imagine opening your armpits and pressing the deepest part of your armpit forward. Keep the shoulders down away from your ears and your upper trapezius (on top of your shoulders) muscles relaxed. Then, slide the shoulder blades up and down on your back 5x.

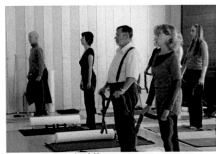

At Hips

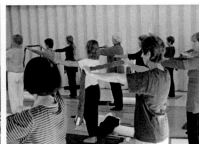

At Collarbones

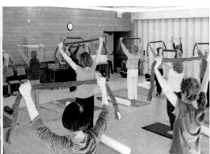

Overhead

Quadruped or Plank: Place the heels of your hands on the towel just under your shoulders, press the palm where your fingers attach to the floor so that your hand slopes down towards the fingers. Hold the shoulder blades wide on your back and arms in a parenthesis shape with elbows slightly bent and creases of the elbow facing each other. Pull gently apart and feel the outside of your armpits working to hold your shoulders wide on your back.

Fletcher Towels may be ordered online for $40 at www.fletcherpilates.com

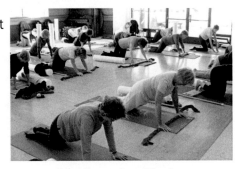

Quadruped or Plank

Sherri R. Betz, PT, GCS, CEEAA, PMA®-CPT
920-A 41st Avenue Santa Cruz, CA 95062 831.476.3100
www.TheraPilates.com

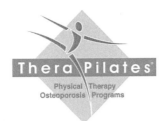

MAT WORK
Foam Roller: Snow Angels

Mounting Safely

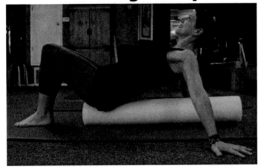

Neutral Spine—Start

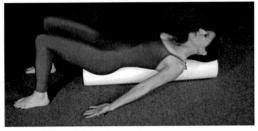

45-90° Chest Stretch

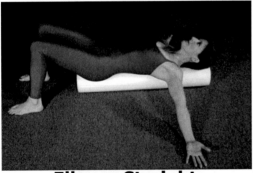

**Elbows Straight-
Fingertips on Floor**

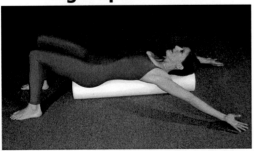

MOUNTING SAFELY
Sit beside Foam Roller with buttocks in line with the very end of the roller.
Lean back on your hands and place one hand with fingers pointing backwards on the opposite side of the roller.
Keep chest lifted and spine in neutral and lift hips up and place the sacrum on the roller.
Carefully slide hands directly apart and lie down on the foam roller.

EXERCISE

Body Position
Neutral spine with head, mid back and convex aspect of sacrum in contact with the roller.
Hands resting at sides.

Movement
Begin by sliding arms with palms up into shoulder abduction.
Stop when you can no longer maintain contact with the floor

Breathing
Prepare with inhalation
Exhale as the shoulders abduct
Inhale as you return to the starting position

Cueing
Axial elongation
Scapular Depression
Rib Depression
Width of chest and upper back
Ease in neck and shoulders

MODIFICATIONS
Body Position
Prop head if increased kyphosis is present
Use towel or yoga mat to cushion roller
Use soft foam roller (888) 330-7272

WATCH FOR
Scapular Elevation
Cervical Extension
Ribs Flaring
Elbow Bending

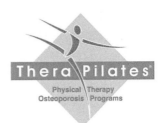

MAT
Foam Roller-90-90° Pelvic Tilt & Leg Lowering

Neutral Spine—Start

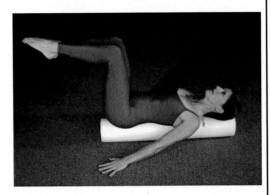

90-90 Gentle Pelvic Tilt

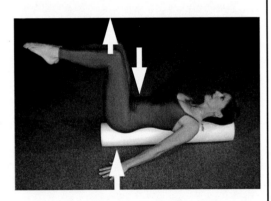

Leg Lowering in Lumbar Neutral on Roller

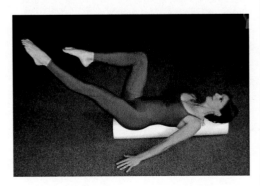

SETUP
Sit beside Foam Roller with buttocks in line with the very end of the roller
Lean back on your hands and place one hand with fingers pointing backwards on the opposite side of the roller
Keep chest lifted and spine in neutral and lift hips up and place the sacrum on the roller
Carefully slide hands directly apart and lie down on the foam roller

Body Position
Neutral spine with head, mid back and convex aspect of sacrum in contact with the roller
Hands resting at sides

EXERCISE
Movement
Begin by bringing knees & hips to 90° angles one at a time keeping abdominal wall firm and carefully maintaining neutral spine
Press the lumbar spine gently into the roller, lifting knees & coccyx 1" up toward the ceiling
Maintain the 90-90 angles of hips and knees throughout movement

Breathing
Prepare with inhalation
Exhale during the posterior pelvic tilt
Inhale as you release to the starting position

Cueing
"Press your knees and tailbone to the ceiling"
Manually pull the patient's knees toward the ceiling
Width of chest and upper back
Avoid pressing back of head into the roller
Ease in the neck and shoulders
Use thick strap under 3rd lumbar vertebrae to check for lumbar spine contact with roller.

VARIATION
Leg Lowering:
As you exhale, extend your knee and point it towards the place where the ceiling meets the wall. Only lower the leg if you can keep your lumbar spine in neutral or if desired, in contact with the roller. Progress to extending leg until it is parallel to the floor with lumbar spine in neutral or flatback.

WATCH FOR
Scapular Elevation
Cervical or Lumbar Extension
Ribs Flaring
Loss of Pelvic Position or Abdominal Bulge

Sherri R. Betz, PT, GCS, CEEAA, PMA®-CPT
920-A 41st Avenue Santa Cruz, CA 95062
831.476.3100   www.TheraPilates.com

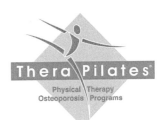

MAT
Foam Roller-

Neutral Spine—Rolling

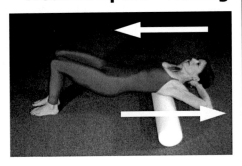

Thoracic Extension

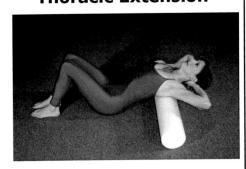

SETUP
Sit with buttocks centered in front of Foam Roller.
Place your hands behind the foam roller with your fingers
  pointed back.
Lean back on your hands.
Keep chest lifted and spine in neutral and carefully slide
hands directly apart.
When your mid-thoracic spine contacts the foam roller,
  immediately place your hands behind your head and keep
  your buttocks resting on the floor.
Body Position
Start in neutral spine with mid back resting against roller
  and hands behind the suboccipital region to
  support the neck.
Elbows wide and ribs engaged with pelvis.

EXERCISE
Movement
Begin rolling back and forth over the thoracic spine only.
Do not roll into the lumbar spine-this is usually painful!
Maintain neutral spine and abdominal contraction
  throughout movement.
Breathing
Prepare with inhalation.
Exhale as the roller moves closer to your feet.
Inhale as the roller moves closer to your head.
Cueing
Draw lowest ribs toward pelvis and keep eyes on ceiling.
Avoid pulling head forward and keep shoulders down.

THORACIC EXTENSION:
Movement
As you roll over the thoracic spine, notice where you
  have tension or sore spots"
When you find one, stop at that segment and place your
  buttocks on the floor
Inhale and extend your thoracic spine over the roller
  without losing the engagement of the ribs with the
pelvis. If the segment is too painful work above and
below it. Exhale and return to the neutral position
Repeat 5-6 times and roll up to the next segment.
Or just work your way slowly up the spine at each
  segment.

WATCH FOR
Scapular Elevation
Cervical or Lumbar Extension
Ribs Flaring
Chin jutting towards the ceiling
Buttocks lifting off the floor

MAT
8" Ball Thoracic Extension

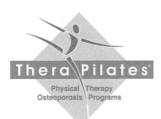

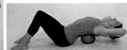

Lower Thoracic Extension

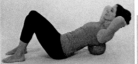

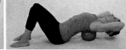

Middle Thoracic Extension

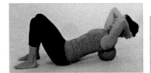

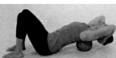

Upper Thoracic Extension

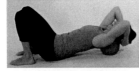

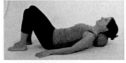

Cervical: Suboccipital Release

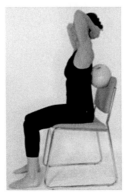

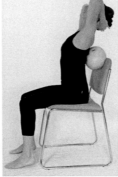

Thoracic Extension Seated in Chair

SETUP
Sit with buttocks centered in front of 8" Air-Filled Ball
Lean back on your hands
Keep chest lifted and spine in neutral and carefully slide
   hands directly apart
When your mid-thoracic spine contacts the ball,
   immediately place your hands behind your head to
   support your neck and keep your buttocks resting on the
   floor

Body Position
Start in a neutral spine with midback resting on the ball
   and hands behind the suboccipital region to support and
   lengthen the neck
Keep elbows wide and ribs engaged with pelvis

EXERCISE
Movement
Begin rolling back and forth over the thoracic spine only.
Do not roll into the lumbar spine-this is usually painful
   and can be damaging!
Maintain neutral spine and mild abdominal contraction
   throughout rolling movement.
As you roll over the thoracic spine, notice where you
   have tension or "sore spots."
When you find one, stop at that segment and place your
   buttocks on the floor.
Inhale and extend your thoracic spine over the ball
   without losing the engagement of the ribs with the
   pelvis.
Exhale and return to the neutral position. Repeat 5-6
times and roll up to the next segment. Or just work your
way slowly up the spine at each segment.

Breathing
Inhale to melt back over the ball as if you are wrapping
your spine around the ball
Exhale, allowing the ribs to descend to return
Imagine that your sternum is like a see-saw on top of
the ball

WATCH FOR
Pulling head forward
Rounding the upper back like a "crunch"
Scapular elevation
Cervical or lumbar extension
Ribs flaring
Chin jutting towards the ceiling
Buttocks lifting off the floor

Sherri R. Betz, PT, GCS, CEEAA, PMA®-CPT
920-A 41st Avenue Santa Cruz, CA 95062
831.476.3100   www.TheraPilates.com

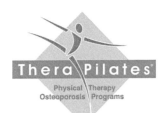

Thera Pilates®
Physical Therapy
Osteoporosis Programs

MAT WORK
Swan Preparation

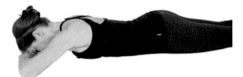

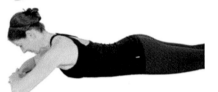

Upper Thoracic Extension

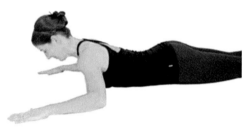

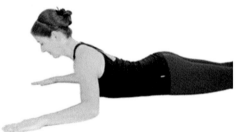

Mid-Thoracic Extension

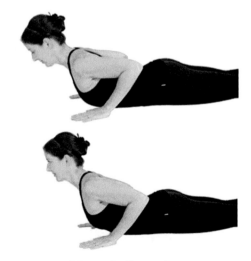

Lower Thoracic Extension

BODY POSITION
Begin with head resting on back of hands in elongated spine position scapulae away from ears. Follow progression below moving from one position to the next.

Upper Thoracic:
Lift head off of mat without changing cervical curve or scapular position *For Strength: Lift hands/forearms off the mat bringing back of hands to touch forehead for strengthening back extensors. Repeat 10x or hold 10 counts*

Mid-Thoracic:
While lifted, open arms to goal post position with 90° abduction and 90° elbow flexion and continue to extend thoracic spine without changing cervical, lumbar or pelvic position.
For Strength: Lift forearms off the mat in goal post position without scapular elevation for strengthening back extensors. Repeat 10x

Lower Thoracic: While lifted, move hands so that fingers are aligned under clavicles, keeping elbows aimed toward feet. Keep pubic bone down.
Extend thoracic spine as far as possible, keeping lowest ribs on the mat without changing cervical, scapular, lumbar or pelvic position
For Strength: Lift hands off the mat at least 1" with no change in torso position to strengthen back extensors. Repeat 10x

MOVEMENT/BREATHING
Inhale to lengthen the spine
Exhale and move into thoracic extension.

WATCH FOR
Watch for head lifting, shoulder elevation, lumbar extension and/or anterior pelvic tilt

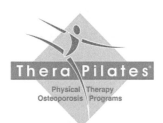

MAT WORK
Swan

Perform Swan Preparation before Full Swan:
Emphasize Mid-Thoracic Extension

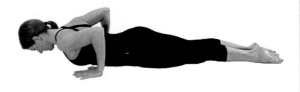

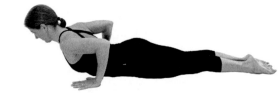

Pre-Swan: Move Hands back 6"

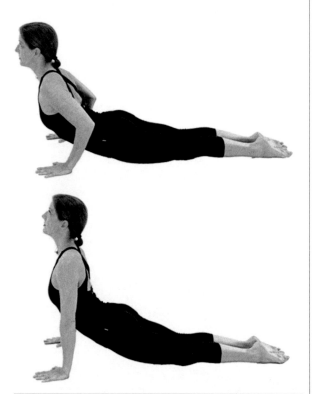

Full Swan: At top, when elbows are straight, hands should be directly under shoulders.

BODY POSITION

Prone, wrists even with lowest ribs, elbows elbows bent, looking straight down, scapulae depressed, neutral spine/pelvis, reaching long with legs, axial elongation.

MOVEMENT / BREATHING

Inhale and reach out through the crown of your head, lift sternum up as you draw the armpits toward the hips, press your hands into the mat as if to "commando crawl" 1" forward, pull your sternum through the frame of your arms, bring scapulae down and back, thoracic spine into extension, keeping pubis in contact with floor, lowest ribs drawing downward, lower abdominals engaged. Keep lowest ribs in contact with the mat as long as possible. Look down at your fingernails to keep cervical spine elongated

Exhale and return to starting position

FULL SWAN VARIATION

If you press the elbows straight keep a posterior tilt of the pelvis and abdominals drawn in to limit lumbar extension. Gaze straight forward.

WATCH FOR

Sagging in the lumbar spine
Hyperextension of neck and lumbar spine
Scapular elevation

Sherri R. Betz, PT, GCS, CEEAA, PMA®-CPT
920-A 41st Avenue Santa Cruz, CA 95062
831.476.3100   www.TheraPilates.com

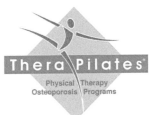

Physical Therapy
Osteoporosis Programs

MAT WORK
Book Opening
(Gentle Thoracic Mobilization)

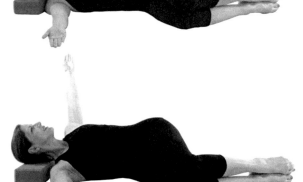

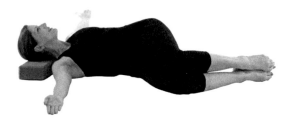

Keep Back Arm Hovering Off Floor

BODY POSITION
Start sidelying with knees bent in neutral
spine.
Pelvis, knees and feet stacked.
Shoulders stacked with hands palm to
palm at 90 deg. Shoulder flexion.
Pillow under head.

MOVEMENT/BREATHING
Inhale to reach the top arm up. Keeping
arm in line with collarbones, begin to exhale
and rotate spine with the arm.
Rotate spine gently as far as possible
keeping pelvis and legs stacked and still.
Hover back arm above the floor. Inhale at
the end of range.
Exhale return arm and spine to stacked
position.
Inhale to return top arm down.
Follow hand with the eyes.

VARIATION
Circle the arm overhead, inhale as the arm
circles up and spine rotates and exhaling as
the arm circles down and around with the
spine returning to neutral position.

WATCH FOR
Rotation of pelvis or sliding of knees.
Flaring of ribs
Pain in the spine
Cervical extension
Shoulder Elevation
Humeral head coming forward.

Sherri R. Betz, PT, GCS, CEEAA, PMA®-CPT
920-A 41st Avenue Santa Cruz, CA 95062
831.476.3100   www.TheraPilates.com

NOTES

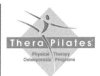
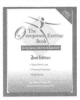

The Osteoporosis Exercise Book: Building Better Bones, 2nd Edition was written to help you incorporate safe mat exercises into your bone-building program. The exercises will help build bone density of the spine and hip, improve posture, balance, flexibility and mobility from beginner to the advanced level exerciser. Learn to avoid movements that increase the risk of fracture. Includes photos, nutritional recommendations, fracture prevention and some of the latest research findings on Osteoporosis.   Over 100 photos, 104 pages. *By Sherri R. Betz, PT*

TheraPilates® Mat for Bone Building & injuries DVD Updated Mat Program based on the latest research and specifically designed for osteoporosis or osteopenia. Incorporate safe and effective Pilates-based Mat exercises to target bone and muscle strength! Safe and challenging exercises target the bones of the spine hips and wrists. Includes Standing Posture and Balance exercises, Fletcher Towelwork®, Foam Roller and 8" Massage Ball exercises, Abdominal Strengthening without Flexion.   *57 minutes*

Yoga for Osteoporosis DVD was based on the latest research with carefully selected poses for osteoporosis or osteopenia. Incorporate safe and effective Yoga poses to improve bone and muscle strength! Learn to modify your yoga practice with the best selection of poses designed for those with bone loss. Safe and challenging poses target the bones of the spine, hips and wrists. Includes: Balancing Poses, Standing & Posture Poses, Leg & Spine Strengthening Poses, Sun Salutation Modifications, Savasana & Meditation.
57 minutes

Pilates Exercises for Osteoporosis DVD was designed by physical therapist, Sherri Betz to help you incorporate safe Pilates exercises into your bone building program. Many Pilates exercises can be unsafe and contraindicated for those with low bone density. By modifying the wonderful exercises of Joseph Pilates and incorporating sound PT principles, you will learn the best exercises to build the bones of the most vulnerable areas of the hip & spinal vertebrae.   *57 minutes*

Pilates for Seniors: The Osteoporosis Workout DVD was developed for Seniors or those who have difficulty getting up and down from the floor for exercises. Explanation of anatomy, proper breathing, spine positioning and deep abdominal contraction precedes the workout. All exercises done in seated or standing position. Includes instructions for safely getting down to and up off the floor without risk for fracture and a few exercises suggestions for exercises that can be done in bed.   *64 minutes*

Prenatal Pilates DVD was developed by Sherri Betz, Physical Therapist, using guidelines from the American College of Obstetrics and Gynecology.   Introduction to proper breathing, spine alignment, transversus abdominus contractions, diastasis recti, and abdominal anatomy followed by a prenatal mat class. All 3 Trimester modifications are demonstrated with precautions and contraindications for a safe workout.
1 Hour 22 mins

Dealing with Acute Low Back Pain DVD was developed by Harry Benich, MPT, to enhance the progress & effectiveness of a physical therapy program for patients with Acute Low Back Injuries. Due to shrinking health insurance reimbursement, PTs are often limited in the time they have with patients and often the treatment programs cannot be completed, restoring patients to full pre-injury status. Included are several principles and basic skills that most patients with spine/lumbo-pelvic injuries should learn to prevent further injury and allow rapid healing to occur!   *55 minutes*

Pre-Pilates for Rehabilitation DVD was designed to introduce you to the Pilates principles of breathing, spinal alignment, core control, shoulder girde alignment, postural re-education, and overall body awareness. Let us help you exercise without increasing your pain. Featuring Sherri Betz, PT and Michele Franzella, PMA®-CPT.   *40 minutes*

Pilates Reformer for Osteoporosis DVD was designed especially for Pilates devotees who have osteoporosis or osteopenia. Included are safe and challenging exercises that target the bone of the spine, hips and wrists. Bone safe practices intro begins the DVD. Great Reformer Selections Include: Footwork with Variations, The Sleeper, Abdominal Strengthening without Flexion, Flowing Long Stretch Series movement sequences. Enjoy your newfound balance, posture, alignment and core control!   *66 minutes*

Page Left Intentionally Blank

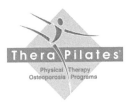

1. THE OSTEOPOROSIS EXERCISE BOOK, 2nd Ed.
2. THERAPILATES® MAT FOR BONE BUILDING DVD
3. YOGA FOR OSTEOPOROSIS DVD
4. PILATES FOR OSTEOPOROSIS DVD
5. THERAPILATES FOR SENIORS DVD
6. PRENATAL PILATES DVD
7. DEALING WITH ACUTE LOW BACK PAIN DVD
8. PRE PILATES FOR REHABILITATION DVD
9. REFORMER FOR OSTEOPOROSIS DVD

Name:_____

Organization:_____

Shipping Address:_____

City:_____State:_____Zip/Postal Code:_____

Phone Home:_____Work:_____

Cell Phone:_____Email Address:_____

Number of Osteoporosis Books :	_____	x 19.95 =	_____
Number of TheraPilates Mat DVD's:	_____	x 24.95 =	_____
Number of Yoga for Osteoporosis DVD's:	_____	x 24.95 =	_____
Number of Osteoporosis DVD's:	_____	x 24.95 =	_____
Number of Senior DVD's:	_____	x 24.95 =	_____
Number of Prenatal DVD's:	_____	x 24.95 =	_____
Number of Low Back Pain DVD's:	_____	x 24.95 =	_____
Number of Pre-Pilates DVD's:	_____	x 24.95 =	_____
Number of reformer DVD's:	_____	x 24.95 =	_____

                    8.5% Tax (CA):   _____

Shipping & Handling- $6 for 1-2 items $12 for 3 or more items:
WHOLESALE PRICE (ANY 12 ITEMS $12.50 EACH)   _____

                              Total: $_____

VISA or MASTERCARD #_____ - _____ - _____ - _____
Expiration Date_____
Name on Card_____
Billing Address _____
City_____State_____Zip Code_____

Or send Check or Money Order Payable to: *TheraPilates*
                                             920-A 41st Avenue
                                             Santa Cruz, CA 95062

Page Left Intentionally Blank

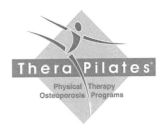

Evaluation:

Please write 3 things you found valuable about this course:

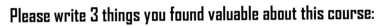

Please write 3 suggestions or things you would like to change about this course:

Please write 3 expectations, goals, skills or information that you would like to gain from this course:

Page Left Intentionally Blank

Title: Intro to TheraPilates® for Bone Building & Injuries
Presenter: Sherri R. Betz, PT, GCS, CEEAA, PMA®-CPT

RELEASE & WAIVER

I, _____ voluntarily desire to participate in physical and rehabilitation and/or exercise training classes conducted by TheraPilates Studio located at: 920-A 41st Avenue Santa Cruz, CA 95062 and understand and agree to the following:

1. I assume full responsibility while voluntarily participating in a training class at my sole risk and shall abide by any rules and regulations for use of the Facility which may be promulgated from time to time by its owner or TheraPilates.

2. I am aware that there exists the possibility of certain conditions occurring during or following training and/or exercise. These include, but are not limited to: mild light headedness, fainting, abnormalities of blood pressure or heart rate, ineffective heart function and in rare instances, heart attack or stroke. The reaction of the cardiovascular system to such activity cannot be predicated with complete accuracy.

3. It is strongly recommended that I receive a medical clearance from my private physician prior to starting an exercise training program. This program is not designed for persons with known heart disease with or without functional impairment.

4. I expressly agree that I have been informed that the program involves possible risks and all exercises shall be undertaken at my sole risk and that neither TheraPilates, nor the Facility at which the program is being conducted, nor the officers, directors, employees or agents of either shall be liable to me nor any other person, for any claims, demands, injuries, damages, actions or causes of action, whatsoever, to my person or property arising out of or connected to my services, facilities, and exercise classes or the Facility where the same is located, and I do hereby release and discharge TheraPilates and the Facility thereof from all claim, demands, injuries, damages, action, or causes of actions and from all acts of active or passive negligence on the part of TheraPilates or the Facility, their servants, agents or employees.

5. I have been offered a copy of this document.

I HAVE READ THE ABOVE STATEMENT AND UNDERSTAND THE CONDITIONS

Participant's Signature: _____ Date: _____

Witness: _____ Date: _____

Page Left Intentionally Blank

Pre and Post Test Questions for TheraPilates® for Osteoporosis:

1. Bone loss that results in a T-score of -1.8 would fall into which of these categories?
   a. osteoporosis
   b. osteopenia
   c. osteoporotic
   d. skeletal fragility

2. What ratio of women over age 50 are at risk for an osteoporotic fracture?
   a. 1 in 5
   b. 3 in 4
   c. 1 in 2
   d. 1 in 4

3. What ratio of men over age 50 are at risk for an osteoporotic fracture?
   a. 1 in 3
   b. 1 in 4
   c. 1 in 5
   d. 1 in 6

4. If a person has one osteoporotic fracture of the spine, that individual's risk of having another spine fracture in one year increases by how much?
   a. 30%
   b. 50%
   c. 100%
   d. 500%

5. What are the most common fracture sites in the spine?
   a. 74, T5, T6
   b. T6, T7, T8
   c. T10, T11, T12
   d. T7, T12, L5

6. In the 1984 Sinaki & Mikkleson study, subsequent fractures occurred in what percentage of those who performed only extension exercises?
   a. 53%
   b. 67%
   c. 16%
   d. 89%

7. What movements are contraindicated for clients/patients with osteoporosis or osteopenia of the spine?
   a. flexion, extension, sidebending
   b. flexion, sidebending, rotation

c. extension, sidebending, rotation

d. flexion, sidebending, extension

8. Which of the following exercises is safe for the osteoporotic or osteopenic client to perform?
    a. Swan Dive 1
    b. Spine Stretch
    c. Rollup
    d. Hundred

9. The first goal of any program for osteoporosis is to learn:

    a. bone-building exercises
    b. hip hinges
    c. fracture prevention techniques
    d. neutral or optimal spine

10. What are the ways to identify osteoporosis?
    a. thoracic kyphosis-Occiput to Wall Distance
    b. height loss
    c. family history
    d. Rib to Pelvis Distance
    e. all of the above

11. Which of the following Pilates exercises is contraindicated for the person with low bone density?
    a. Open Leg Rocker
    b. Leg Circles
    c. Side Kick
    d. Leg Pull

12. Osteoporosis is a systemic skeletal disease characterized by:
    a. decreased cortical bone
    b. increased trabecular bone
    c. decreased bone fragility
    d. increased bone fragility

13. What is the best type of exercise for osteoporosis?
    a. Weightbearing exercise or weight training
    b. Jumping or Plymetrics (Volleyball, Football, Soccer)
    c. Endurance exercise (Running, cycling, swimming)
    d. Yoga, Pilates and Tai Chi
    e. It depends on the age of the client
    f. It depends on the bone density of the client

Calcium-Rich Foods

Green Leafy Vegetables (1 Cup Cooked)

•Collard greens	350 mg
•Wild Greens	350 mg
•Broccoli	150 mg
•Kale	179 mg
•Spinach	278 mg
•Turnip Greens	229 mg
•Beet Greens	165 mg
•Bok Choy	230 mg
•Mustard Greens	160 mg
•Rhubarb	348 mg
•Parsley (raw)	122 mg
•Dandelion Greens	147 mg
•Okra	220 mg
•Rutabaga	100 mg

Sea Vegetables

•Hijiki	610 mg
•Wakame	520 mg
•Kombu	305 mg
•Agar-Agar (Dry Flakes)	400 mg
•Dulse (Dry)	567 mg
•Nori (1/4 cup)	300 mg

Beans and Legumes (1 cup cooked)

•Tofu-firm (Calcium-sulfate/Cl) 4 oz	400 mg
•Tempeh 4 oz	172 mg
•Garbanzo Beans (chickpeas)	150 mg
•Black Beans	135 mg
•Pinto Beans	128 mg
•Corn Tortilla	60 mg
•Black-eyed Peas	210 mg
•Great Northern Beans	130 mg
•Lima and White Beans	160 mg
•Navy Beans	120 mg
•Soybeans	200 mg

Fish

•Canned mackerel- 3 oz	260 mg
•Perch	115 mg
•Salmon-canned w/bones	200 mg
•Salmon-cooked	130 mg
•Sardines-canned w/ bones	340 mg
•Shrimp-cooked	95 mg
•Oysters	80 mg
•Clams	60 mg
•Lobster-cooked	55 mg

Grains

•Bran Muffin	115 mg
•Corn Bread	115 mg
•Corn Tortilla	60 mg
•Cold Cereal-fortified (average)	250 mg
•Oatmeal-1 cup	20 mg
•Instant Oatmeal-fortified,1 cup	100 mg
•Amaranth-cooked, 1 cup	275 mg
•Quinoa-cooked, 1 cup	80 mg

Nuts and Seeds

Sesame Seeds- 1 oz.	280mg
•Ground sesame seeds (Tahini) 3T	300 mg
•Almonds- 1 cup	200 mg
•Sunflower Seeds- 1 cup hulled	174 mg
•Brazil Nuts- 1 cup	260 mg
•Hazelnuts- 1 cup	282 mg
•Walnuts– 1cup	280 mg
•Soy Nuts (dry roasted)-1 cup	370 mg
•Poppy Seeds- 1 T	125 mg

Mineral Waters

•Perrier	140 mg
•San Pellegrino	200 mg
•Gerolsteiner	300 mg
•Mendocino	380 mg
•Contexeville	451 mg
•Apollinaris (Schweppes)	91 mg
••Evian	78 mg
•Black Mountain	25 mg
•Arrowhead	20 mg
•Fiji Natural Artesian	17 mg
•Crystal Geyser	8.3 mg
•Calistoga	4 mg

Dairy

•Skim Milk 1 cup	300 mg
•Nonfat yogurt 1 cup	294 mg
•Low fat cottage cheese	150 mg

Other Sources of Calcium

•Blackstrap Molasses 1 T	137 mg
•Orange juice, fortified	210 mg
•Rice Milk, fortified	240 mg
•Soy Milk, fortified	160 mg
•Dried Figs- 5 medium	135 mg

Herbs
•Kukicha (Twig Tea- 6x Ca+ of Milk!)
•Yellow dock leaves/roots
•Dandelion leaves/roots
•Plantain leaves
•Nettle leaves
•Raspberry leaves/canes/berries
•Mugwort leaves
•Red Clover blossoms

Used with Permission from Christiane Northrup's Women's Bodies, Women's Wisdom

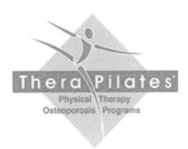

Sherri's Osteogenic Salad!
Eat every day!!

Arugula
Carrot Sticks
Broccoli
Sliced Apples
White Mushrooms
Cherry Tomatoes
Canned Chickpeas
Canned Beets
Grated Parmesan or Romano Cheese
Tamari Roasted Almonds
Fresh Dill
Fresh Parsley
1 cup Cooked Brown Rice
Toasted Sesame Oil
Marukan Rice Wine Vinegar (Yellow Label)
Or Nakano Rice Wine Vinegar (Original Flavor Red Label)

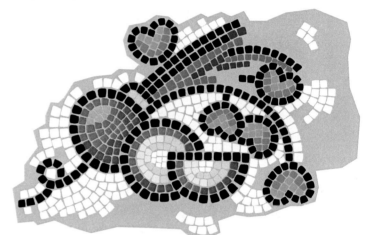

Toss all items, sprinkle with Sesame Oil and Rice Wine Vinegar and enjoy!

Since the research shows that the protective effects on bone produced by vegetables, salads, and herbs are not merely due to their metabolic alkalinity, scientists are now theorizing that the bone-boosting effects are due to pharmacologically active compound(s) in the herbs and vegetables. Future research will undoubtedly uncover the compounds responsible, but fortunately, we don't have to wait to reap the bone-saving benefits. All we need to do is enjoy lots of onions, garlic, parsley, dill, tomatoes, cucumbers and green leafy salads.
References:

Muhlbauer RC, Li F. Effect of vegetables on bone metabolism. *Nature* 1999 Sep 23;401(6751):343-4.

Muhlbauer RC, Lozano A, Reinli A. Onion and a mixture of vegetables, salads, and herbs affect bone resorption in the rat by a mechanism independent of their base excess. *J Bone Miner Res* 2002 Jul;17(7):1230-6.

Vitamin & Mineral Suggested Supplementation

B VITAMINS

Thiamine B_1	100 mg
Riboflavin	10 mg
Niacin B	130 mg
Niacinamide	30 mg
Pantothenic Acid B_5	450 mg
Pyridoxine B_6	50 mg
Cobalamin B_{12}	250 mg
Folic Acid	2 mg

C, D, E VITAMINS

Beta Carotene	25,000 IU
Vitamin C	2000 mg
Vitamin D3	400-2000 IU
Vitamin E (d-alpha tocopherol)	400 IU

MINERALS

Calcium (Citrate or Malate)	1200-1500 mg
Magnesium	600-750 mg
Potassium	90 mg
Zinc-Picolinate	15-25 mg
Manganese Picolinate	15 mg
Boron Picolinate	2-6 mg
Copper	1 mg
Chromium	150-200 mcg
Selenium picolinate	100-200 mcg
Molybdenum picolinate	100 mcg
Vanadium picolinate	100 mcg

Recommended by Christiane Northrup, MD

NOTES

Page Left Intentionally Blank

42174813R00034

Made in the USA
San Bernardino, CA
28 November 2016